I0693526

# ACID REFLUX COOKBOOK FOR SENIORS

*A Senior's Guide to Comforting Nutrient-Rich Recipes to Soothe Acid Reflux Symptoms*

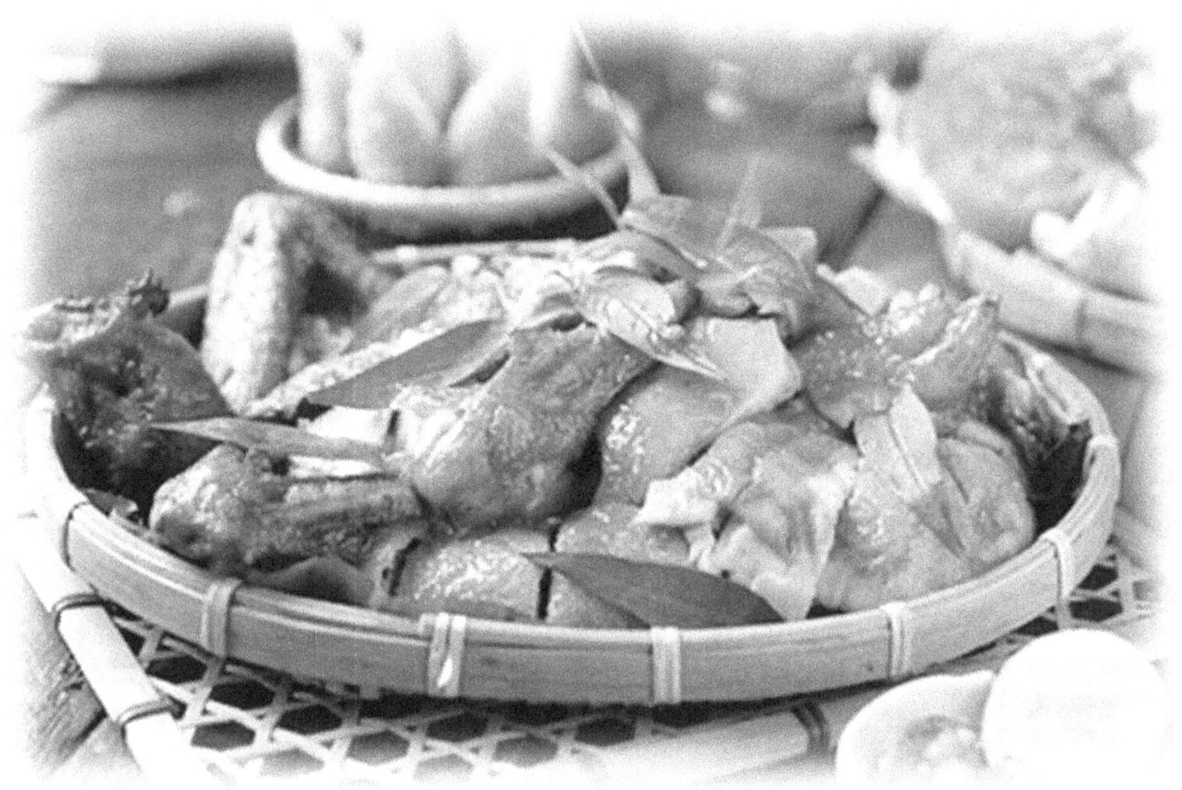

## CHRISTIANA WHITE

**Copyright © 2024 Christiana White**

All rights reserved. No part of this publication may be reproduced, distributed, or transmitted in any form or by any means, including photocopying, recording, or other electronic or mechanical methods, without the prior written permission of the publisher, except in the case of brief quotations embodied in critical reviews and certain other non-commercial uses permitted by copyright law.

GAIN ACCESS TO MORE BOOKS

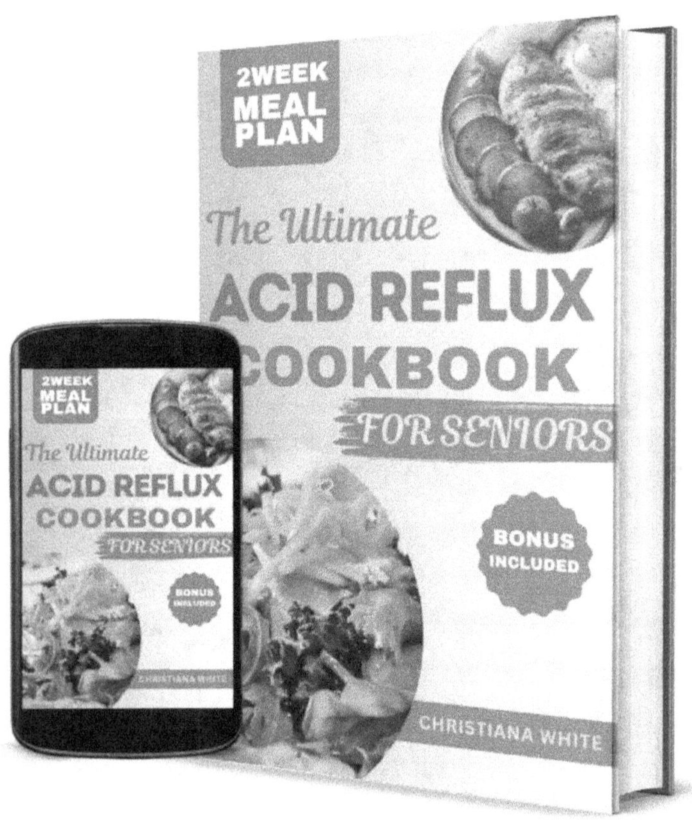

# TABLE OF CONTENTS


INTRODUCTION .................................................................................. 7

Understand Acid Reflux in Seniors ....................................... 9

Diet Is Important for Managing Acid Reflux. ...................... 10

How Can This Cookbook Help? .......................................... 10

CHAPTER 1 ..................................................................... 12

What Is Acid Reflux? ......................................................... 12

The Causes and Triggers of Acid Reflux in Seniors .......... 12

Symptoms & Complications ............................................... 14

CHAPTER 2 ..................................................................... 15

Seniors' Guide to the Acid Reflux Diet ............................. 15

Principles of the Acid Reflux Diet for Seniors ................. 15

Foods To Avoid. ................................................................. 16

Foods to Include ................................................................. 17

The Significance of Portion Control and Meal Timing ...... 17

CHAPTER 3 ..................................................................... 19

Breakfast Recipes ............................................................... 19

Oatmeal with Sliced Banana .............................................. 19

Banana Pancakes (Low Fat Version) .................................. 20

Ginger-Infused Herbal Tea ................................................. 21

Baked Apples with Cinnamon. ....................................................... 22

Chia Seed Pudding ..................................................................... 23

Scrambled Tofu with Spinach ...................................................... 24

Whole-Grain Toast with Almond Butter. ...................................... 25

Blueberry Smoothie (non-citrus). ................................................ 26

Quinoa Porridge and Ripe Peaches............................................... 27

Warm Rice Pudding (With Almond Milk) ..................................... 28

CHAPTER 4 ................................................................................ 29

Lunch And Dinner Recipes:......................................................... 29

Baked Sweet Potatoes with Fennel. .............................................. 29

Broccoli and Brown Rice Stir-fry ................................................ 30

Lettuce Wraps with Lean Chicken ............................................... 31

Quinoa Stuffed Bell Peppers........................................................ 33

Chickpea Salad with Cucumber and Dill ...................................... 34

Zucchini Noodles (Zoodles) With Tomato Sauce........................... 35

Miso Glazed Eggplant ................................................................. 36

Cauliflower Mash........................................................................ 37

Turkey and Vegetable Soup ......................................................... 38

Salmon Fillet and Steamed Asparagus ......................................... 40

CHAPTER 5 ................................................................................ 41

Snacks & Light Bites ............................................................... 41

Melon Salad (Watermelon, Cantaloupe, And Honeydew) ........................ 41

Celery with Cucumber Sticks ...................................................... 42

Almond Butter with Whole-Grain Crackers ...................................... 43

Rice Cakes with Avocado Slices .................................................. 44

Herbal Infusions: Chamomile, Peppermint, Ginger ............................. 45

Carrot Sticks and Hummus ........................................................ 46

Baked Sweet Potato Fries (Lightly Seasoned) ................................... 47

Pear Slices with Almond Ricotta. ................................................. 48

Cherry Tomatoes and Basil ........................................................ 49

Pumpkin seeds (pepitas). .......................................................... 50

CHAPTER 6 .......................................................................... 51

Beverages ........................................................................... 51

Chamomile Tea ..................................................................... 51

Aloe Vera Juice (diluted) .......................................................... 52

Coconut Water ...................................................................... 53

Filtered Water with Lemon Slices. ................................................ 53

Green Tea (decaffeinated) ......................................................... 54

Golden Milk (Turmeric Latte) ..................................................... 55

Ginger Tea (warm or iced) ......................................................... 56

Herbal Infusions (Licorice Root, Lemon Balm)......................................................... 57

Non-Citrus Fruit Smoothies (Banana, Papaya, Spinach) ........................... 58

Fresh Mint Tea ........................................................................................ 59

CHAPTER 7 .............................................................................................. 60

Desserts ................................................................................................... 60

Banana "Nice Cream" (A Frozen Banana Dessert) ..................................... 60

Baked Apples with Cinnamon. ................................................................. 61

Chia Seed Pudding with Berries .............................................................. 62

Pumpkin Custard (With Almond Milk) ...................................................... 63

Coconut Rice Pudding (Lightly sweetened) ............................................... 64

Baked Pear Halves with Cinnamon and Walnuts. ...................................... 65

Avocado Chocolate Mousse (No Added Sugars) ........................................ 66

Date and Walnut Energy Bites. ................................................................. 67

Rice Cake With Almond Butter and Dark Chocolate Chips. ....................... 68

Berry Parfait (Layered Yogurt with Berries and Granola) .......................... 69

CHAPTER 8 .............................................................................................. 70

Bonus....................................................................................................... 70

2-Week Meal Plan..................................................................................... 70

CONCLUSION ........................................................................................... 75

# INTRODUCTION

Welcome to the Acid Reflux Cookbook for Seniors, your go-to guide for managing GERD, heartburn, and acid reflux symptoms with nutrition. This book contains a revolutionary journey that will help you restore comfort, vigor, and joy in your daily life.

For many seniors, the struggle with acid reflux can overshadow even the most modest joys. The discomfort, the sleepless nights, the restrictions on what you can eat--it can feel like a continuous battle. But don't worry, you have a beacon of hope, a road plan to relief.

Over the years, this cookbook has become a treasured companion for elders like you, providing not just recipes but also a lifeline to a more pleasant life. We've curated a range of foods that will relax your digestive system, alleviate your discomfort, and excite your taste buds.

Imagine waking up in the morning, not to the gnawing pain of heartburn, but to the aroma of a delicious, reflux-friendly meal waiting for you. Consider eating large, fulfilling meals throughout the day, knowing that each bite is nourishing your body and promoting your health. Consider gathering with loved ones and sharing meals without fear or uncertainty, knowing you have the tools to handle any eating circumstance with ease.

This book is more than a cookbook; it is a lifeline, a source of empowerment, and a tribute to the human spirit's tenacity. It serves as a reminder that no matter what hurdles we face, there is always a way forward, and that with the appropriate guidance and support, we can conquer even the most tenacious of obstacles.

Whether you've had acid reflux for years or are just starting out on your path to relief, this book is for you. It's a promise that you're not alone, that there's hope, and that better days are ahead.

So, to all the seniors out there who have felt the grip of acid reflux tighten around their lives, I invite you to take a leap of faith, to believe in the power of food as medicine, and to embark on this path to a brighter, more comfortable tomorrow. Your body deserves it, your spirit needs it, and with this cookbook as a guide, you can make it happen.

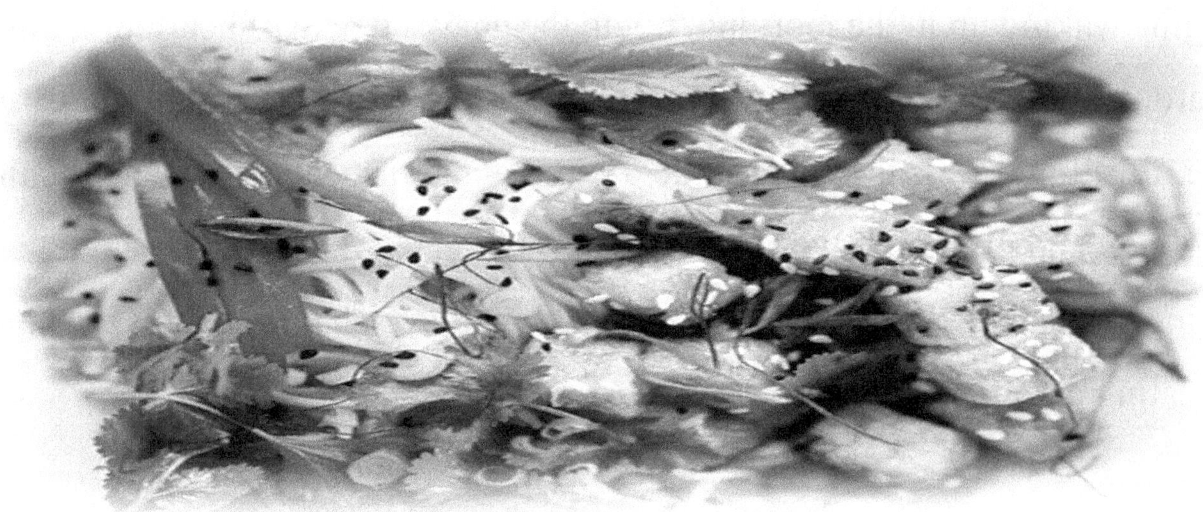

## _Understand Acid Reflux in Seniors_

Acid reflux, also known as gastroesophageal reflux disease (GERD), is a common digestive illness that strikes elderly more frequently than younger people. It occurs when the stomach's acidic contents run backward into the esophagus, causing irritation, inflammation, and pain.

Seniors are more vulnerable to acid reflux due to a variety of factors including age-related changes in the digestive system, weakening esophageal muscles, and other medical disorders.

Many seniors experience acid reflux symptoms such as heartburn, regurgitation of sour liquid or food, difficulty swallowing, and, in some cases, persistent coughing or hoarseness. Left untreated, acid reflux can progress to more serious consequences like esophagitis, Barrett's esophagus, and even esophageal cancer.

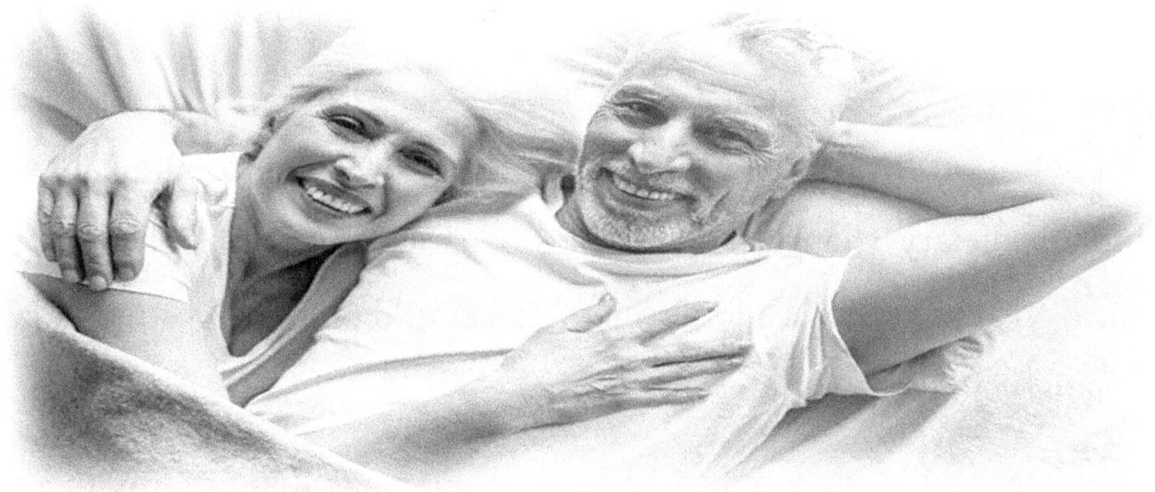

## *Diet Is Important for Managing Acid Reflux.*

Diet is an important factor in treating acid reflux for elders. Certain meals and beverages might cause or worsen symptoms, whilst others can assist relieve pain and encourage healing.

Seniors who make strategic food choices can considerably reduce the frequency and intensity of acid reflux episodes, resulting in a higher quality of life and general well-being.

The key elements of an acid reflux diet for seniors are to avoid acidic and spicy foods, fatty and fried foods, coffee, chocolate, alcohol, and carbonated beverages. Instead, seniors are recommended to eat a mix of low-acid, high-fiber foods such fruits, vegetables, lean meats, whole grains, and non-acidic dairy products. It's also important to practice portion control, eat smaller, more frequent meals, and avoid lying down just after eating.

## *How Can This Cookbook Help?*

This cookbook is an invaluable resource for seniors wishing to alleviate acid reflux through dietary changes. It provides a varied range of delicious and healthy meals that are specifically designed to be mild on the digestive system while yet satisfying the appetite.

Each recipe is carefully prepared to include components that are low in acid, easy to digest, and high in critical nutrients. This cookbook includes everything from warm breakfast alternatives to nourishing soups and salads, hearty main dishes, and seductive desserts, ensuring that seniors never have to trade flavor for digestive comfort.

Furthermore, this cookbook includes practical suggestions, meal planning tactics, and lifestyle guidelines to help seniors manage their acid reflux efficiently. Whether you're a seasoned cook or new to the kitchen, whether you're dining alone or throwing a party, this cookbook enables seniors to take control of their health and live a life free of the misery of acid reflux.

In essence, this cookbook is more than a collection of recipes; it is a complete reference, a source of inspiration, and a beacon of hope for seniors dealing with acid reflux. Seniors can use this cookbook to help them improve their digestive health, feel better, and enjoy more delicious food.

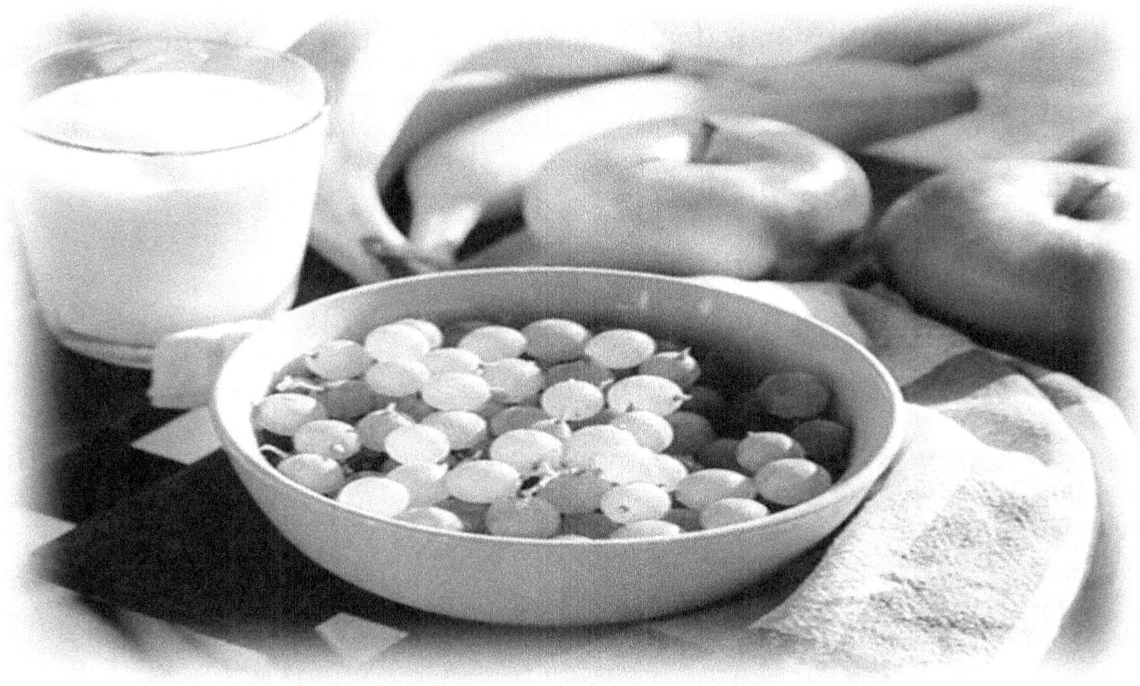

# CHAPTER 1

## *What Is Acid Reflux?*

Acid reflux, also known as gastroesophageal reflux disease (GERD), is a persistent digestive ailment in which stomach acid backflows into the esophagus. The esophagus is a tube that links the mouth and stomach. Normally, a ring of muscle at the bottom of the esophagus called the lower esophageal sphincter (LES) relaxes to let food and liquid into the stomach and then tightens to prevent stomach contents from flowing back up into the esophagus.

However, in people who have acid reflux, this process is hampered. The LES can weaken or relax abnormally, allowing stomach acid to pass into the esophagus. This acidic reflux irritates the esophageal lining, causing symptoms such as heartburn, regurgitation of sour liquid or food, chest pain, difficulty swallowing, and a persistent cough.

## *The Causes and Triggers of Acid Reflux in Seniors*

Several factors can contribute to the development or worsening of acid reflux in seniors:

- **Age-Related Changes**: As people age, the muscles that support the LES can weaken, making it less efficient at preventing acid reflux.

- **Hiatal Hernia**: Seniors are more susceptible to hiatal hernias, which occur when a part of the stomach protrudes into the chest cavity via the diaphragm. This can weaken the LES, increasing the likelihood of acid reflux.

- **Medications**: Some medications often provided to seniors, including as nonsteroidal anti-inflammatory drugs (NSAIDs), calcium channel blockers, and sedatives, can relax the LES or irritate the esophagus, causing acid reflux.

- **Obesity**: Excess weight, especially around the midsection, puts pressure on the stomach, which can push stomach contents up into the esophagus.

- **Dietary Factors**: Eating large meals, fatty or fried foods, spicy foods, citrus fruits, tomatoes, chocolate, coffee, and alcohol can cause or worsen acid reflux in seniors.

- **Smoking**: Tobacco use weakens the LES and increases stomach acid production, aggravating acid reflux symptoms.

- **Other Medical disorders:** Seniors with underlying medical disorders such as hiatal hernias, gastroparesis, or scleroderma are more likely to experience acid reflux.

- Heartburn is a burning sensation in the chest that typically happens after eating or at night.
- Regurgitation: A sour liquid or food that comes back up into the throat or mouth.
- Difficulty Swallowing: The sensation of food stuck in the throat or chest.
- Chronic cough: Consistent coughing, especially during night.
- Hoarseness or sore throat: Acid reflux can irritate the vocal cords.
- Chest Pain: Discomfort or pain in the chest, which is frequently misinterpreted for heart attack.

**If not managed, acid reflux can cause issues such as:**

- Esophagitis is inflammation or irritation of the esophageal lining.
- Barrett's Esophagus is a precancerous condition in which the cells lining the esophagus alter as a result of persistent acid exposure.
- Esophageal Stricture: A narrowing of the esophagus caused by scarring from frequent acid exposure.
- Respiratory Issues: Acid reflux can worsen asthma symptoms or cause aspiration pneumonia if stomach contents are inhaled into the lungs.

Seniors with acid reflux symptoms should seek medical attention and appropriate treatment to avoid complications and improve their quality of life. Furthermore, making lifestyle adjustments, such as changing your food, can help relieve symptoms and lessen the frequency of acid reflux.

# CHAPTER 2

## _Seniors' Guide to the Acid Reflux Diet_

Dietary modifications have a major impact on the frequency and severity of acid reflux symptoms. This chapter delves into the basics of an acid reflux diet for seniors, concentrating on foods to avoid and include, as well as the need of portion control and meal planning.

## _Principles of the Acid Reflux Diet for Seniors_

- **Limit Acidic Foods:** Although stomach acid is necessary for digestion, too much acid can irritate the esophagus, creating heartburn. The goal is to lower the total acid load in the stomach.
- **Limit Fatty and Spicy Foods:** Fatty and spicy foods can relax the lower esophageal sphincter (LES), which is the muscle valve that keeps stomach contents from spilling back up.
- **Improve Digestion**: Certain foods and lifestyle behaviors can help food move more efficiently through the digestive tract, minimizing the amount of time stomach acid can irritate the esophagus.

- **Citrus Fruits and Juices:** Grapefruits, oranges, lemons, and tomatoes are strong in acidity and can aggravate acid reflux symptoms.
- **Chocolate and peppermint:** These relax the LES, allowing stomach acid to increase.
- **Fatty Foods:** Fried foods, fatty cuts of meat, and processed meats are hard to digest and can put strain on the LES.
- **Spicy meals,** such as chili peppers and curries, might irritate the esophagus.
- **Peppermint and spearmint:** These relax the LES, which worsens reflux.
- **Garlic and onions:** Although some people tolerate them, they can irritate the esophagus in others.
- **Caffeine and alcohol**: Both can irritate the esophagus while relaxing the LES.
- **Carbonated beverages:** The fizz can irritate the esophagus and distend the stomach, putting additional strain on the LES.

## Foods to Include

- **Low-Acid Fruits and Vegetables:** Bananas, melons, pears, green beans, broccoli, and leafy greens are low in acidity and contain critical nutrients.

- **Ginger**: Ginger contains anti-inflammatory qualities that may benefit the esophagus.

- **Lean Protein:** Skinless chicken, fish, and beans provide protein without the fat that might cause reflux.

- **Whole Grains:** Brown rice, quinoa, and whole wheat bread promote digestion and provide long-lasting energy.

- **Healthy Fats:** Olive oil and avocado contain vital fats without aggravating reflux.

- **Non-Citrus Fruits:** Bananas, melons, and pears are low in acidity and provide essential vitamins and minerals.

## The Significance of Portion Control and Meal Timing

- Smaller, More Frequent Meals: Eating smaller meals throughout the day minimizes stomach distention and puts less pressure on the LES.

- Avoid Eating Late at Night: Having a full stomach when lying down increases the chance of reflux. Aim for a light dinner at least three hours before bed.

- Chew thoroughly to improve digestion and lessen the workload on the stomach.

**Additional Considerations:**

- **Individual Triggers**: Certain foods can cause reflux in some seniors but not others. It's critical to understand and prevent personal triggers.

- **Hydration**: Staying hydrated might help reduce stomach acid and aid digestion. Aim for water throughout the day.

- **Weight Management:** Excess weight can put strain on the abdomen and aggravate reflux. Keeping a healthy weight might be advantageous.

- **Consult a doctor or Dietitian:** A doctor or certified dietitian can design a personalized acid reflux diet plan based on your unique needs and health concerns.

Seniors who follow these suggestions and consult with a healthcare practitioner can effectively manage acid reflux and live a more pleasant and healthy lifestyle.

# CHAPTER 3

*Breakfast Recipes*

## *Oatmeal with Sliced Banana*

- ***Serves: 1***
- ***Prep time: 10 minutes.***

**Ingredients*:***

- One cup of heated oatmeal.
- 8 ounces of skim or dairy-free milk.
- 1/2 cup fresh papaya, cubed
- 1/2 banana, sliced
- Two pieces of whole wheat bread.
- 1 tablespoon of your preferred spread or butter.

**Instructions:**

- Prepare the oatmeal according to the package directions.
- Add in the skim or dairy-free milk.
- Combine the cubed papaya and sliced banana.
- Serve with whole-wheat toast topped with butter or a dairy-free option.

**Nutritional values (per serving):**

- *Calories: About 350 kcal*
- *Fiber: 6 g.*

- *Protein: 10 g.*

## Banana Pancakes (Low Fat Version)

- **Servings: two.**
- **Prep time: 15 minutes.**

**Ingredients:**

- One ripe banana.
- 2 eggs
- 1/4 teaspoon of vanilla extract.
- One-quarter teaspoon baking powder
- Cooking spray or a little oil for the pan.

**Instructions:**

- Mash a ripe banana in a bowl.
- Combine the egg, vanilla essence, and baking powder. Mix well.
- Heat a nonstick skillet over medium heat, then lightly coat with cooking spray or oil.
- Pour little amounts of batter into the skillet to produce pancakes.
- Cook until bubbles appear on the surface, then flip and cook the opposite side.
- Serve warm, topped with cinnamon or honey.

**Nutritional values (per serving):**

- *Calories: About 180 kcal*
- *Protein: 7 g.*
- *Fat: 6 g.*

## *Ginger-Infused Herbal Tea*

- **Serves: 1**
- **Prep time: 5 minutes.**

**Ingredients:**

- One cup of boiling water.
- 1 inch of fresh ginger root, peeled and sliced
- Optional: honey or lemon for flavoring

**Instructions:**

- Bring the water to a boil, then add the ginger slices.
- Allow it to steep for 5 minutes.
- Strain the tea into a cup.
- If preferred, add honey or lemon.

**Nutritional values (per serving):**

- *Calories: Around 5 kcal*
- *No fat or protein.*
- *Ginger contains anti-inflammatory properties.*

## _Baked Apples with Cinnamon._

- *Servings: two.*
- *Prep time: 10 minutes.*

## Ingredients:

- 2 medium apples (sweet types, such as Fuji or Honeycrisp).
- One teaspoon of ground cinnamon.
- 1 tablespoon of chopped pecans (optional).
- 1 teaspoon coconut oil, melted

## Instructions:

- Preheat the oven to 350°F/175°C.
- Core the apples and remove the seeds, but keep the bottoms intact.
- Combine melted coconut oil and ground cinnamon.
- Coat the inside of each apple with the cinnamon-coconut oil mixture.
- Arrange the apples in a baking dish and top with chopped pecans (if using).
- Bake for 30 to 40 minutes, or until the apples are soft.
- Serve warm for a satisfying breakfast or dessert.

## Nutritional values (per serving):

- *Calories: Around 120 kcal*
- *Fiber: 4 grams.*
- *The natural sweetness of apples helps satiate appetites.*

## _Chia Seed Pudding_

- **_Servings: two._**
- **_Preparation time: 5 minutes, including chilling time._**

## Ingredients:

- 1/4 cup of chia seeds.
- One cup unsweetened almond milk.
- 1 tablespoon maple syrup (optional; adjust to taste).
- Fresh berries (blueberries and raspberries) for topping.

## Instructions:

- In a bowl, combine the chia seeds and almond milk. Stir thoroughly to mix.



- If you like it sweeter, add maple syrup.
- Refrigerate for at least 2 hours, or overnight, to allow the chia seeds to absorb the liquid.
- Serve chilled and topped with fresh berries.

## Nutritional values (per serving):

- _Calories: Around 120 kcal_
- _Fiber: 8 g._
- _Chia seeds include omega-3 fatty acids, which enhance heart health._

# <u>*Scrambled Tofu with Spinach*</u>

- *Servings: two.*
- *Prep time: 15 minutes.*

## Ingredients:

- 1 block (14 oz) of crumbled extra-firm tofu
- 2 cups fresh spinach leaves.
- One tablespoon of olive oil.
- 1/2 teaspoon of turmeric powder.
- Add salt and pepper to taste.

## Instructions:

- Heat olive oil in a nonstick skillet over medium heat.
- Add the crushed tofu and simmer for 5 minutes, stirring periodically.
- Sprinkle the turmeric powder, salt, and pepper over the tofu.
- Add fresh spinach leaves and simmer until wilted.
- Serve warm for a protein-rich breakfast.

## Nutritional values (per serving):

- *Calories: About 150 kcal*
- *Protein: 12 g.*
- *Iron-rich tofu and spinach promote general wellness.*

## *Whole-Grain Toast with Almond Butter.*

- *Serves: 1*
- *Prep time: 5 minutes.*

## Ingredients:

- One piece of whole grain bread (gluten-free if necessary)
- 1 tablespoon almond butter, unsweetened
- Optional: sliced banana or berries for topping.

## Instructions:

- Toast the whole grain bread till golden brown.
- Spread the almond butter evenly over the toast.
- Optional: top with sliced banana or berries.
- Enjoy this simple and filling meal!

## Nutritional values (per serving):

- *Calories: Around 200 kcal*
- *Fiber: 4 grams.*
- *Almond butter contains healthy fats, which give satiety.*

## _Blueberry Smoothie (non-citrus)._

- ***Serves: 1***
- ***Prep time: 5 minutes.***

### Ingredients:

- One cup unsweetened almond milk.
- One-half cup frozen blueberries
- One ripe banana.
- One spoonful of chia seeds.
- Optional: 1 teaspoon of honey (adjust to taste).

### Instructions:

- In a blender, mix almond milk, frozen blueberries, banana, and chia seeds.
- Blend until smooth and creamy.
- Taste and add honey as needed for sweetness.
- Serve in a chilled glass.

### Nutritional values (per serving):

- Calories: Around 200 kcal
- Fiber: 7 grams.
- Antioxidants found in blueberries promote overall health.

## *Quinoa Porridge and Ripe Peaches*

- ***Servings: two.***
- ***Prep time: 15 minutes.***

**Ingredients:**

- One cup cooked quinoa.
- Two ripe peaches, peeled and sliced
- One tablespoon of honey (optional)
- 1/4 teaspoon of ground cinnamon.
- 1/4 cup of unsweetened almond milk.

**Instructions:**

- In a bowl, combine the cooked quinoa, sliced peaches, honey (if using), and ground cinnamon.
- Mix thoroughly to equally spread the flavors.
- Drizzle with unsweetened almond milk.
- Serve either warm or cooled.

**Nutritional values (per serving):**

- Calories: Around 200 kcal
- Fiber: 5 g.
- Protein: 6 g.

## _Warm Rice Pudding (With Almond Milk)_

- _**Servings: two.**_
- _**Prep time: 20 minutes.**_

**Ingredients:**

- One cup of cooked brown rice.
- One cup unsweetened almond milk.
- One tablespoon of maple syrup.
- 1/2 teaspoon of vanilla extract.
- Ground nutmeg for garnish.

**Instructions:**

- In a saucepan, combine the cooked brown rice, almond milk, maple syrup, and vanilla essence.
- Heat over low-medium heat, stirring often, until the liquid thickens (approximately 15 minutes).
- Serve warm, dusted with a pinch of grated nutmeg.

**Nutritional values (per serving):**

- _Calories: About 180 kcal_
- _Fiber: 3 grams._
- _Creamy and comforting._

<h1 style="text-align:center">CHAPTER 4</h1>



*Lunch And Dinner Recipes:*

*Baked Sweet Potatoes with Fennel.*

- ***Servings: two.***
- ***Prep time: 10 minutes.***

## Ingredients:

- Two medium sweet potatoes.
- 1 small fennel bulb, finely sliced
- One tablespoon of olive oil.
- Add salt and pepper to taste.

## Instructions:

- Preheat your oven to 400°F (200°C).
- Scrub the sweet potatoes and pierce with a fork.
- Place the sweet potatoes on a baking pan and bake for 45–50 minutes, or until soft.
- While the sweet potatoes bake, sauté the sliced fennel in olive oil until softened.
- Slice open the cooked sweet potatoes, fluff the flesh with a fork, and top with the sautéed fennel.
- Season with salt and pepper.

**Nutritional values (per serving):**

- *Calories: About 180 kcal*

- *Fiber: 6 g.*

- *Fennel contains vitamin C, which helps immune function.*

## *Broccoli and Brown Rice Stir-fry*

- ***Servings: four.***

- ***Prep time: 15 minutes.***

**Ingredients:**

- One cup brown rice.

- 1 lb. of broccoli florets. Þ

- 1 red bell pepper, thinly sliced

- 1 carrot julienned

- 2 garlic cloves, minced[4]

- Two teaspoons low-sodium soy sauce.

- One tablespoon of olive oil.

- One teaspoon of grated fresh ginger.

**Instructions:**

- Cook the brown rice according to the package instructions.

- Heat olive oil in a large skillet or wok over medium-high heat.

- Sauté minced garlic and grated ginger for 1 minute.

- Combine the broccoli florets, red bell pepper, and julienned carrot. Stir-fry for approximately 5-7 minutes, or until vegetables are tender-crisp.
- Stir in the cooked brown rice and soy sauce. Throw everything together.
- Serve hot for a tasty and healthful stir-fry.

**Nutritional values (per serving):**

- *Calories: About 250 kcal*
- *Protein: 8 g.*
- *Fiber: 6 g.*

## *Lettuce Wraps with Lean Chicken*

- ***Servings: two.***
- ***Prep time: 20 minutes.***

**Ingredients:**

- 1 pound of lean ground chicken.
- 1 small onion, coarsely chopped
- 2 garlic cloves, minced
- One red bell pepper, chopped
- 1 grated carrot.
- One tablespoon of olive oil.
- Two teaspoons low-sodium soy sauce.
- One teaspoon of honey.

- Boston or Bibb lettuce leaves for wrapping.

**Instructions:**

- Heat the olive oil in a skillet over medium heat.
- Combine the chopped onion and minced garlic. Sauté till fragrant.
- Add the ground chicken and heat until browned.
- Mix in the chopped bell pepper, grated carrot, soy sauce, and honey. Cook for a couple further minutes.
- Wash and separate the lettuce leaves.
- Fill the lettuce leaves with the chicken mixture.
- Serve as a refreshing lettuce wrap.

**Nutritional values (per serving):**

- *Calories: About 280 kcal*
- *Protein: 25 g.*
- *Carrots include vitamin A, which helps eye health.*

<u>*Quinoa Stuffed Bell Peppers*</u>

- ***Servings: two.***
- ***Prep time: 20 minutes.***

## Ingredients:

- Two large bell peppers, either red, yellow, or green
- One cup cooked quinoa.
- 1/2 cup of diced tomatoes.
- 1/2 cup of cooked black beans.
- 1/4 cup of chopped fresh parsley.
- 1/4 teaspoon ground cumin.
- Add salt and pepper to taste.

## Instructions:

- Preheat your oven to 375°F (190°C).
- Cut off the tops of the bell peppers and remove the seeds.
- In a bowl, combine cooked quinoa, diced tomatoes, black beans, chopped parsley, ground cumin, salt, and pepper.
- Stuff the bell peppers with quinoa mixture.
- Arrange the filled peppers in a baking dish and cover with aluminum foil.
- Bake for 30–35 minutes, or until the peppers are soft.
- Serve warm for a nutritious and tasty supper.

**Nutritional values (per serving):**

- *Calories: About 250 kcal*

- *Fiber: ten grams.*

- *Protein: 12 g.*

## *Chickpea Salad with Cucumber and Dill*

- ***Servings: two.***

- ***Prep time: 15 minutes.***

**Ingredients:**

- 1 can (15 oz) of drained and rinsed chickpeas

- One medium cucumber, diced

- 1/4 cup freshly chopped dill.

- Two teaspoons of extra virgin olive oil.

- One tablespoon of lemon juice.

- Add salt and pepper to taste.

**Instructions:**

- In a bowl, combine chickpeas, diced cucumber, and dill.

- Drizzle with olive oil and lemon juice.

- Season with salt and pepper.

- Toss everything until thoroughly blended.

- Serve chilled as a refreshing salad.

**Nutritional values (per serving):**

- *Calories: About 280 kcal*

- *Fiber: ten grams.*

- *Olive oil contains healthy fats that support heart health.*

## *Zucchini Noodles (Zoodles) With Tomato Sauce.*

- **Servings: two.**

- **Prep time: 15 minutes.**

**Ingredients:**

- Two medium zucchinis spiralized into noodles (zoodles).

- 1 cup tomato sauce, low-acid kind

- 1 clove garlic, minced

- One tablespoon of olive oil.

- Fresh basil leaves as garnish

**Instructions:**

- Heat the olive oil in a skillet over medium heat.

- Sauté for 1 minute with minced garlic.

- Add the zucchini noodles and simmer for 2-3 minutes, until cooked.

- Pour the tomato sauce over the zoodles and mix well.

- Serve warm and garnish with fresh basil leaves.

**Nutritional values (per serving):**

- *Calories: About 150 kcal*

- *Fiber: 4 grams.*

- *Low-acid tomato sauce lowers reflux risk.*

## *Miso Glazed Eggplant*

- ***Servings: two.***

- ***Prep time: 20 minutes.***

**Ingredients:**

- One large eggplant chopped into rounds.

- Two teaspoons of white miso paste.

- One tablespoon low-sodium soy sauce.

- One tablespoon of honey (adjust to taste).

- One teaspoon of grated fresh ginger.

- 1 clove garlic, minced

- One tablespoon of olive oil.

**Instructions:**

- Preheat your oven to 400°F (200°C).

- In a separate bowl, combine white miso paste, soy sauce, honey, grated ginger, and minced garlic to make the glaze.

- Coat both sides of the eggplant slices in olive oil.

- Arrange the eggplant rounds on a baking sheet and brush with the miso glaze.
- Bake the eggplant for 15-20 minutes, or until soft and caramelized.
- Serve warm as a delicious side dish.

**Nutritional values (per serving):**

- *Calories: Around 120 kcal*
- *Fiber: 5 g.*
- *Miso contains probiotics and promotes intestinal health.*

## *Cauliflower Mash*

- ***Servings: two.***
- ***Prep time: 15 minutes.***

**Ingredients:**

- 1 medium head cauliflower, chopped into florets.
- 2 garlic cloves, minced
- Two teaspoons of olive oil.
- Add salt and pepper to taste.

**Instructions:**

- Steam or boil cauliflower florets until soft.
- In a separate skillet, cook the minced garlic in olive oil until aromatic.
- Place the cooked cauliflower and sautéed garlic in a food processor.

- Blend until smooth and creamy.

- Season with salt and pepper.

- Serve as a tasty alternative to mashed potatoes.

**Nutritional values (per serving):**

- *Calories: Around 100 kcal*

- *Fiber: 5 g.*

- *Low in carbohydrates and mild on the stomach.*

## *Turkey and Vegetable Soup*

- ***Servings: four.***

- ***Prep time: 20 minutes.***

**Ingredients:**

- 1 pound of cooked turkey (leftover or roasted), shredded

- 4 cups of reduced sodium chicken or veggie broth

- 2 cups chopped veggies (carrots, celery, green beans, and zucchini)

- 1 onion, diced

- 2 garlic cloves, minced

- One teaspoon dried thyme.

- Add salt and pepper to taste.

## Instructions:

- In a large pot, cook diced onion and minced garlic until tender.
- Add the chopped mixed vegetables and simmer for a few minutes.
- Add the chicken or vegetable broth and bring to a simmer.
- Combine shredded turkey and dried thyme.
- Simmer for 15-20 minutes, until the vegetables are soft.
- Season with salt and pepper.
- Serve warm for a cozy and nutritious soup.

## Nutritional values (per serving):

- *Calories: About 250 kcal*
- *Protein: 25 g.*
- *High in vitamins and minerals.*

*Salmon Fillet and Steamed Asparagus*

- *Servings: two.*
- *Prep time: 20 minutes.*

## Ingredients:

- Two salmon fillets.
- 1 bunch asparagus, trimmed
- One lemon, cut
- Two teaspoons of olive oil.
- Add salt and pepper to taste.

## Instructions:

- Preheat your oven to 375°F (190°C).
- Arrange the salmon fillets on a baking pan lined with parchment paper.
- Arrange the asparagus around the fish.
- Drizzle olive oil on the fish and asparagus.
- Season with salt and pepper.
- Garnish with lemon slices.
- Bake for 15-20 minutes, or until the salmon is cooked thoroughly.
- Serve hot for a light, heart-healthy meal.

## Nutritional values (per serving):

- *Calories: About 300 kcal*
- *Omega-3 fatty acids found in salmon promote general wellness.*

# CHAPTER 5

*<u>Snacks & Light Bites</u>*

*<u>Melon Salad (Watermelon, Cantaloupe, And Honeydew)</u>*

- ***Servings: two.***
- ***Prep time: 10 minutes.***

**Ingredients:**

- 1 cup watermelon, cubed
- 1 cup cubed cantaloupe.
- 1 cup honeydew melon, cubed
- Fresh mint leaves as garnish

**Instructions:**

- In a large bowl, combine the watermelon, cantaloupe, and honeydew melon.
- Gently mix the melon cubes together.
- Garnish with fresh mint leaves.
- Serve chilled for a refreshing and hydrating snack.

**Nutritional values (per serving):**

- *Calories: Around 60 kcal*

- *Vitamin C from melon promotes immunological function.*

- *Hydrating and low-fat*

## Celery with Cucumber Sticks

- ***Servings: two.***

- ***Prep time: 5 minutes.***

**Ingredients:**

- Cut 2 celery stalks into sticks.

- 1 cucumber, peeled and chopped into sticks

- Hummus for dips

**Instructions:**

- Arrange the cucumber and celery sticks on a platter.

- Serve with a side of hummus to dip.

- Enjoy this crispy, hydrating snack.

**Nutritional values (per serving):**

- *Calories: About 30 kcal*

- *Fiber: 2g*

- *Low in calories and refreshing.*

## _Almond Butter with Whole-Grain Crackers_

- *Servings: two.*
- *Prep time: 2 minutes.*

**Ingredients:**

- Four full grain rice cakes or crackers.
- Two tablespoons of almond butter.
- Sliced banana (optional).

**Instructions:**

- Spread almond butter equally over each rice cake or cracker.
- Optional: top with sliced banana.
- Enjoy this well-balanced snack that contains healthy fats and fiber.

**Nutritional values (per serving):**

- *Calories: About 150 kcal*
- *Protein: 4 grams.*
- *Healthy fats from almond butter.*

## *Rice Cakes with Avocado Slices*

- ***Servings: two.***
- ***Prep time: 5 minutes.***

## Ingredients:

- Two whole grain rice cakes.
- One ripe avocado, sliced
- One pinch of sea salt.
- Optional: a sprinkling of red or black pepper flakes

## Instructions:

- Transfer the whole-grain rice cakes to a platter.
- Garnish each rice cake with slices of ripe avocado.
- Add a pinch of sea salt to the avocado.
- If preferred, season with black pepper or red pepper flakes.
- Enjoy this simple and tasty snack that is easy on the stomach.

## Nutritional values (per serving):

- *Calories: About 150 kcal*
- *Healthy fats from avocados*
- *Fiber from whole grain rice cakes.*

- ***Serving Size: 1 cup per infusion.***
- ***Preparation time is 5 minutes (plus steeping time).***

## Ingredients:

- One teaspoon of dried chamomile flowers.
- One teaspoon of dried peppermint leaves.
- One teaspoon of dried ginger slices.
- One cup of boiling water.

## Instructions:

In a teapot or cup, mix together the dried chamomile, peppermint, and ginger.
- Pour boiling water over the herbs.
- Cover and simmer for 5-8 hours (or overnight) to let the flavors infuse.
- Strain the infusion into a cup.
- Take a sip carefully and enjoy the calming benefits of these herbal infusions.

## Nutritional values (per serving):

- *Calories: Negligible (mostly herbal benefits)*
- *Chamomile: Calms and helps digestion.*
- *Peppermint: Improves digestion and reduces bloating.*
- *Ginger is anti-inflammatory and helps with nausea alleviation.*

<u>*Carrot Sticks and Hummus*</u>

- ***Servings: two.***
- ***Prep time: 10 minutes.***

## Ingredients:

- 2 large carrots peeled and sliced into sticks.
- 1/2 cup hummus, either store-bought or homemade.

## Instructions:

- Arrange carrot sticks on a platter.
- Serve with a side of hummus to dip.
- Enjoy this crispy, fiber-rich snack that is easy on your tummy.

## Nutritional values (per serving):

- *Calories: Around 100 kcal*
- *Fiber: 4 grams.*
- *Carrots include beta-carotene, which helps general health.*

<u>*Baked Sweet Potato Fries (Lightly Seasoned)*</u>

- ***Servings: two.***
- ***Prep time: 10 minutes.***

## Ingredients:

- Peel two medium sweet potatoes and chop them into fries.
- One tablespoon of olive oil.
- A pinch of sea salt.
- Optional: Sprinkle with paprika or cayenne pepper.

## Instructions:

- Preheat your oven to 400°F (200°C).
- Season the sweet potato fries with olive oil, sea salt, and optional seasonings.
- Spread them on a baking sheet.
- Bake for 20-25 minutes, or until light brown and crispy.
- Savor these guilt-free and tasty fries.

## Nutritional values (per serving):

- Calories: About 150 kcal
- Vitamin A from sweet potatoes promotes immune health.

<u>*Pear Slices with Almond Ricotta.*</u>

- ***Servings: two.***
- ***Prep time: 10 minutes.***

## Ingredients:

- One ripe pear, thinly cut
- 1/2 cup almond ricotta, store-bought or homemade.
- Drizzle with natural honey.

## Instructions:

- Place the pear slices on a platter.
- Garnish each piece with a dollop of almond ricotta.
- Drizzle with natural honey.
- Enjoy this sweet and creamy snack that is easy on your stomach.

## Nutritional values (per serving):

- Calories: About 150 kcal
- Fiber: 4 grams.
- Almond ricotta contains plant-based protein.

## *Cherry Tomatoes and Basil*

- ***Servings: two.***
- ***Prep time: 5 minutes.***

## Ingredients:

- One cup of cherry tomatoes.
- Fresh basil leaves.
- A pinch of sea salt.

## Instructions:

- Wash and cut the cherry tomatoes in half.
- Arrange tomato halves on a platter.
- Tear the fresh basil leaves and spread them over the tomatoes.
- Season with a pinch of sea salt.
- Savor this simple yet tasty snack.

## Nutritional values (per serving):

- Calories: About 30 kcal
- Vitamin C from tomatoes promotes immunological function.

## *Pumpkin seeds (pepitas).*

- *Servings: two.*
- *Prep time: 5 minutes.*

**Ingredients:**

- 1/2 cup pepitas (raw pumpkin seeds)
- A pinch of sea salt.
- Optional: Sprinkle with paprika or cayenne pepper.

**Instructions:**

- Preheat the oven to 350°F/175°C.
- Mix the pumpkin seeds with a teaspoon of sea salt and optional spices.
- Spread them on a baking sheet.
- Roast for 10–12 minutes, or until gently golden.
- Allow to cool and enjoy as a crunchy and nutritious snack.

**Nutritional values (per serving):**

- *Calories: About 150 kcal*
- *High in magnesium and zinc.*

# CHAPTER 6



## *Chamomile Tea*

- ***Serving Size: 1 cup***
- ***Prep time: 5 minutes.***

**Ingredients:**

- One chamomile tea bag or a teaspoon of dried chamomile flowers
- One cup of boiling water.
- Optional: honey or lemon for flavoring

**Instructions:**

- Put a chamomile tea bag or dried chamomile flowers in a cup.
- Pour boiling water over the teabag or flowers.
- Steep for around 5 minutes to infuse the flavors.
- To enhance the flavor, add honey or lemon juice.
- Drink carefully and enjoy the soothing properties of chamomile.

**Nutritional values (per serving):**

- *Calories: Negligible (mostly herbal benefits)*
- *Soothing and mild for the stomach*

## _Aloe Vera Juice (diluted)_

- ***Serving Size: 1 cup***
- ***Prep time: 2 minutes.***

## Ingredients:

- 1/4 cup pure aloe vera juice, diluted with 3/4 cup water.
- Optional: a little honey for sweetness.

## Instructions:

- Add water to the aloe vera juice to dilute it.
- If preferred, add a small amount of honey.
- Serve cold or room temperature.
- Aloe vera may calm the esophagus and improve digestive health.

## Nutritional values (per serving):

- Calories: Around 10 kcal.
- Hydrating and beneficial to digestion.

## *Coconut Water*

- *Serving Size: 1 cup*
- *Preparation time: 0 minutes (ready to drink).*

**Ingredients:**

- 1 cup natural coconut water (without added sugar)

**Instructions:**

- Just pour the coconut water into a glass.
- Serve chilled or on ice.
- Coconut water is both refreshing and hydrating.

**Nutritional values (per serving):**

- Calories: Around 45 kcal
- Contains electrolytes and potassium.


## *Filtered Water with Lemon Slices.*

- ***Serving size: 1 glass.***
- ***Prep time: 2 minutes.***

**Ingredients:**

- One glass filtered water.
- Slices of fresh lemon

**Instructions:**

- Fill a glass of filtered water.
- Include a few slices of fresh lemon.
- Allow a few minutes to infuse the water with lemon taste.
- Enjoy this refreshing and hydrating drink throughout the day.

**Nutritional values (per serving):**

- *Calories: Negligible (mostly hydration benefits).*
- *Lemons include vitamin C and antioxidants.*


## *Green Tea (decaffeinated)*

- ***Serving Size: 1 cup***
- ***Prep time: 5 minutes.***

**Ingredients:**

- One decaffeinated green tea bag.
- One cup of boiling water.

**Instructions:**

- Place the green tea bag into a cup.
- Pour boiling water over the tea bag.
- Allow it to steep for 3–5 minutes.
- Remove the tea bag and enjoy this calming, antioxidant-rich beverage.

**Nutritional values (per serving):**

- Calories: Negligible (mostly antioxidant benefits)
- Green tea promotes digestive and general health.

## *Golden Milk (Turmeric Latte)*

- ***Serving Size: 1 cup***
- ***Prep time: 5 minutes.***

**Ingredients:**

- 1 cup of unsweetened almond milk (or other non-dairy milk).
- 1/2 teaspoon of ground turmeric.
- 1/4 teaspoon of ground cinnamon.
- One sprinkle of black pepper.
- For sweetness, add honey or maple syrup.

**Instructions:**

- In a small saucepan, heat the almond milk over low heat.
- Combine the ground turmeric, cinnamon, and black pepper.
- Optional: sweeten with honey or maple syrup.
- Pour into a cup and enjoy this soothing, anti-inflammatory drink.

**Nutritional values (per serving):**

- *Calories: About 40 kcal*
- *Turmeric contains curcumin, a compound recognized for its health benefits.*

## *Ginger Tea (warm or iced)*

- **Serving Size: 1 cup**
- **Prep time: 5 minutes.**

**Ingredients:**

- One cup of water.
- 1 inch of fresh ginger root, peeled and sliced
- Optional: honey or lemon for flavoring

**Instructions:**

- Heat the water in a saucepan.
- Boil the water, then add the sliced ginger.
- Allow it to simmer for five minutes.
- Strain the ginger tea into a cup.
- Add honey or lemon to taste.
- Drink this calming, anti-inflammatory beverage.

**Nutritional values (per serving):**

- *Calories: Negligible (mostly herbal benefits)*
- *Ginger may reduce inflammation and relieve acid reflux symptoms.*

## *Herbal Infusions (Licorice Root, Lemon Balm)*

- **Serving Size: 1 cup per infusion.**
- **Preparation time is 5 minutes (plus steeping time).**

**Ingredients:**

- One teaspoon of dried lemon balm leaves.
- One teaspoon of dried licorice root.
- One cup of boiling water.

**Instructions:**

- Put the dried lemon balm and licorice root in a cup.
- Pour boiling water over the herbs.
- Cover and simmer for 5-8 hours (or overnight) to let the flavors infuse.
- Strain the infusion into a cup.
- Drink carefully and enjoy the relaxing benefits of these herbal infusions.

**Nutritional values (per serving):**

- *Calories: Negligible (mostly herbal benefits)*
- *Lemon balm and licorice root may help with digestion and acid reflux problems.*

- ***Servings: One smoothie.***
- ***Prep time: 5 minutes.***

## Ingredients:

- One cup unsweetened almond milk.
- One cup of frozen pineapple pieces.
- 1/2 cup frozen strawberries.
- One ripe banana.
- One cup of fresh spinach.
- One teaspoon of flaxseeds

## Instructions:

- Blend all of the ingredients until smooth.
- If necessary, increase the amount of almond milk to achieve desired consistency.
- Serve chilled for a nutritious, reflux-friendly smoothie.

## Nutritional values (per serving):

- *Calories: About 150 kcal*
- *Fiber: 5 g.*
- *Vitamins and minerals found in fruits and spinach*

## *Fresh Mint Tea*

- ***Serving Size: 1 cup***
- ***Prep time: 5 minutes.***

## Ingredients:

- One cup of boiling water.
- 2-3 sprigs of fresh mint leaves
- Optional: honey or lemon for flavoring

## Instructions:

- Add boiling water to a cup.
- Add the fresh mint leaves.
- Allow it to steep for 3–5 minutes.
- Optional: add honey or lemon.
- Enjoy this delightful and calming mint tea.

## Nutritional values (per serving):

- *Calories: Negligible (mostly herbal benefits)*
- *Mint can aid digestion and add a nice flavor.*

# CHAPTER 7



## *Desserts*

### *Banana "Nice Cream" (A Frozen Banana Dessert)*

- *Servings: two.*
- *Prep time: 10 minutes.*

**Ingredients:**

- Two ripe bananas, peeled and sliced.
- One teaspoon of vanilla extract.
- Optional toppings include chopped nuts, dark chocolate chips, and fresh berries.

**Instructions:**

- Freeze the banana slices for at least two hours.
- In a food processor, combine the frozen banana slices and vanilla extract until smooth.
- Serve immediately as soft-serve, or freeze for a firmer texture.

**Nutritional values (per serving):**

- *Calories: 120.*
- *Fiber: 3 grams.*
- *Sugar: 14 grams.*

## *Baked Apples with Cinnamon.*

- ***Servings: four.***
- ***Prep time: 15 minutes.***

## Ingredients:

- Four medium apples, cored and cut.
- One tablespoon of lemon juice.
- One teaspoon of ground cinnamon.
- One tablespoon of coconut oil (optional).

## Instructions:

- Preheat the oven to 350°F/175°C.
- Combine the apple slices, lemon juice, and cinnamon.
- Place the slices in a baking tray and drizzle with coconut oil (if desired).
- Bake for 25–30 minutes, or until tender.

## Nutritional values (per serving):

- *Calories: 100.*
- *Fiber: 4 grams.*
- *Sugar: 18 grams.*

- ***Servings: two.***

- ***Preparation time: 5 minutes, including chilling time.***

## Ingredients:

- 1/4 cup of chia seeds.

- One cup unsweetened almond milk (or oat milk).

- 1 cup mixed berries, fresh or frozen.

- 1 tablespoon of maple syrup (optional).

## Instructions:

- Combine chia seeds and almond milk in a bowl. Stir well and chill for at least two hours (or overnight).

- Place the chia pudding in serving glasses and top with mixed berries.

- Drizzle with maple syrup if desired.

## Nutritional values (per serving):

- *Calories:180*

- *Fiber: 12 grams.*

- *Sugar: 8 grams.*

## *Pumpkin Custard (With Almond Milk)*

- ***Servings: six.***
- ***Prep time: 10 minutes.***

## Ingredients:

- 1 can (15 oz) of pumpkin puree
- One cup unsweetened almond milk.
- 1/4 cup maple syrup.
- One teaspoon of vanilla extract.
- One teaspoon pumpkin pie spice (or cinnamon and nutmeg)

## Instructions:

- Preheat your oven to 375°F (190°C).
- Combine all ingredients until smooth.
- Pour into individual ramekins and bake for approximately 1 hour and 10 minutes.

## Nutritional values (per serving):

- *Calories: 90.*
- *Fiber: 4 grams.*
- *Sugar: 10 grams.*

<u>*Coconut Rice Pudding (Lightly sweetened)*</u>

- ***Servings: four.***
- ***Prep time: 10 minutes.***

## Ingredients:

- 1 cup cooked white rice, cooled
- 1 can of full-fat coconut milk (13.5 oz)
- 2 tablespoons of maple syrup (adjust to taste).
- 1/2 teaspoon of vanilla extract.
- Optional toppings include toasted coconut flakes and sliced almonds.

## Instructions:

- In a saucepan, mix together the cooked rice, coconut milk, maple syrup, and vanilla essence.
- Cook over low to medium heat, stirring often, until the sauce thickens (approximately 15-20 minutes).
- Remove from heat and allow it cool slightly.
- Serve warm or chilled, garnished with toasted coconut flakes or sliced almonds.

## Nutritional values (per serving):

- *Calories: 250.*
- *Fiber: 2 grams.*
- *Sugar: 10 grams.*

<u>*Baked Pear Halves with Cinnamon and Walnuts.*</u>

- *Servings: two.*
- *Prep time: 10 minutes.*

## Ingredients:

- Two ripe pears, halved and cored
- One teaspoon of ground cinnamon.
- 2 tablespoons of chopped walnuts.
- One tablespoon of honey (optional)

## Instructions:

- Preheat your oven to 375°F (190°C).
- Arrange the pear halves on a baking sheet, cut side up.
- Sprinkle with cinnamon, then top with chopped walnuts.
- Drizzle with honey if desired.
- Bake for 20-25 minutes, until the pears are soft.

## Nutritional values (per serving):

- *Calories: 150.*
- *Fiber: 6 grams.*
- *Sugar: 18 grams.*

## *Avocado Chocolate Mousse (No Added Sugars)*

- ***Servings: two.***
- ***Prep time: 10 minutes.***

**Ingredients:**

- One ripe avocado.
- Two teaspoons of unsweetened cocoa powder.
- One teaspoon of vanilla extract.
- 1/4 cup of unsweetened almond milk.
- Optional toppings include fresh berries and shaved dark chocolate.

**Instructions:**

- Scoop out the avocado flesh and combine with the cocoa powder, vanilla essence, and almond milk until smooth.
- Refrigerate for a minimum of 30 minutes.
- Serve in tiny bowls and garnish with fresh berries or shaved dark chocolate.

**Nutritional values (per serving):**

- *Calories:180*
- *Fiber: 8 grams.*
- *Sugar: 2 grams.*

## *Date and Walnut Energy Bites.*

- ***Serving size: 12 nibbles.***
- ***Prep time: 15 minutes.***

## Ingredients:

- One cup of pitted dates
- One cup of walnuts.
- One spoonful of chia seeds.
- One teaspoon of vanilla extract.
- A pinch of salt.

## Instructions:

- In a food processor, combine the dates, walnuts, chia seeds, vanilla essence, and salt until a sticky consistency forms.
- Form the mixture into little balls (approximately one tablespoon each).
- Refrigerate for at least 30 minutes before serving.

## Nutritional values (per bite):

- *Calories: 90.*
- *Fiber: 2 grams.*
- *Sugar: 9 grams.*

## *Rice Cake With Almond Butter and Dark Chocolate Chips.*

- ***Servings: two.***
- ***Prep time: 5 minutes.***

## Ingredients:

- 2 rice cakes (either whole grain or plain)
- Two tablespoons of almond butter.
- One tablespoon of dark chocolate chips (70% cocoa or higher).

## Instructions:

- Spread almond butter equally over each rice cake.
- Sprinkle the dark chocolate chips on top.
- Enjoy as a crisp and delicious snack.

## Nutritional values (per serving):

- *Calories:180*
- *Fiber: 2 grams.*
- *Sugar: 6 grams.*

## *Berry Parfait (Layered Yogurt with Berries and Granola)*

- ***Servings: two.***
- ***Prep time: 10 minutes.***

**Ingredients:**

- 1 cup plain Greek yogurt (low or nonfat)
- One cup of mixed berries (blueberries, raspberries, strawberries).
- 1/4 cup granola (use a low-sugar option)

**Instructions:**

- In serving glasses, layer the Greek yogurt, mixed berries, and granola.
- Build layers until you reach the top.
- Garnish with additional berries.
- Serve immediately, or chill until ready to eat.

**Nutritional values (per serving):**

- *Calories: 200.*
- *Fiber: 6 grams.*
- *Sugar: 12 grams.*

# CHAPTER 8

*Bonus*

## *2-Week Meal Plan*

**Week 1**

**Day 1**

- Breakfast: oatmeal with sliced bananas.

- Lunch: Baked sweet potatoes with fennel.

- Dinner: Broccoli and Brown Rice Stir-Fry.

- Snack: Melon salad (watermelon, cantaloupe, and honeydew)

- Beverage: Chamomile Tea

**Day 2**

- Breakfast: Banana Pancakes (Low Fat Version)

- Lunch: lettuce wraps with lean chicken.

- Dinner: Cauliflower Mash.

- Snack: Celery and cucumber sticks.

- Drink: Aloe Vera Juice (diluted)

**Day 3**

- Breakfast: Ginger-infused herbal tea.

- Lunch: Turkey and vegetable soup.

- Dinner: salmon fillet with steamed asparagus.

- Snack: Almond butter on whole grain crackers.
- Beverage: Coconut water

## Day 4

- Breakfast: Baked apples with cinnamon.
- Lunch: Quinoa Stuffed Bell Peppers
- Dinner: Chickpea salad with cucumber and dill.
- Snack: Rice cakes with avocado slices.
- Drink: Ginger tea (warm or iced).

## Day 5

- Breakfast: Chia seed pudding.
- Lunch: Zucchini noodles with tomato sauce.
- Dinner: Miso Glazed Eggplant
- Snack: carrot sticks and hummus.
- Drink: Herbal infusions (lemon balm, licorice root).

## Day 6

- Breakfast: scrambled tofu with spinach.
- Lunch: Baked pear halves with cinnamon and walnuts.
- Dinner is Quinoa Porridge with Ripe Peaches.
- Snack: Baked Sweet Potato Fries, lightly seasoned.
- Beverage: non-citrus fruit smoothies (banana, papaya, spinach).

**Day 7**

- Breakfast: Whole-grain toast with almond butter.
- Lunch: Chickpea salad with cucumber and dill.
- Dinner: Zucchini noodles (zoodles) with tomato sauce.
- Snack: Pear slices with almond ricotta.
- Drink: filtered water with lemon slices.


**Week 2**

**Day 8**

- Breakfast: blueberry smoothie (non-citrus).
- Lunch: Salmon Fillet and Steamed Asparagus
- Dinner: Chickpea salad with cucumber and dill.
- Snack: Cherry tomato with basil.
- Drink: Green Tea (Decaffeinated

**Day 9**

- Breakfast: Quinoa porridge with ripe peaches
- Lunch: Quinoa Stuffed Bell Peppers
- Dinner: Miso Glazed Eggplant
- Snack: pumpkin seeds (pepitas).
- Beverage: Turmeric Latte or Golden Milk

**Day 10**

- Breakfast: Warm Rice Pudding (With Almond Milk)

- Lunch: Baked sweet potatoes with fennel.

- Dinner: Broccoli and Brown Rice Stir-Fry.

- Snack: Herbal infusions (chamomile, peppermint, ginger).

- Beverage: Fresh mint tea

## Day 11

- Breakfast: oatmeal with sliced bananas.

- Lunch: lettuce wraps with lean chicken.

- Dinner: Cauliflower Mash.

- Snack: Almond butter on whole grain crackers.

- Drink: Aloe Vera Juice (diluted)

## Day 12

- Breakfast: Banana Pancakes (Low Fat Version)

- Lunch: Turkey and vegetable soup.

- Dinner: salmon fillet with steamed asparagus.

- Snack: Rice cakes with avocado slices.

- Drink: Ginger tea (warm or iced).

## Day 13

- Breakfast: Ginger-infused herbal tea.

- Lunch: Baked pear halves with cinnamon and walnuts.

- Dinner is Quinoa Porridge with Ripe Peaches.

- Snack: Baked Sweet Potato Fries, lightly seasoned.

- Beverage: non-citrus fruit smoothies (banana, papaya, spinach).

**Day 14**

- Breakfast: scrambled tofu with spinach.
- Lunch: Chickpea salad with cucumber and dill.
- Dinner: Zucchini noodles (zoodles) with tomato sauce.
- Snack: Pear slices with almond ricotta.
- Drink: filtered water with lemon slices.

# CONCLUSION

As we near the end of our journey through the Acid Reflux Cookbook for Seniors, it's important to reflect on the significant aspects we've covered and provide words of encouragement and motivation to seniors who manage acid reflux through nutrition.

This book has covered the essentials of acid reflux, including its causes, triggers, symptoms, and potential problems. We've talked about the importance of dietary changes in managing acid reflux for seniors, including foods to avoid and meals to embrace. with breakfast to dinner, snacks to beverages, we've compiled a broad collection of delicious and healthy meals designed exclusively for seniors suffering with acid reflux.

We've also provided practical suggestions and tactics for meal planning, grocery shopping, dining out, and managing social situations, allowing seniors to regain control of their digestive health and live without the misery of acid reflux.

I applaud all of the seniors who have taken the initiative to improve their intestinal health. Managing acid reflux can be difficult, but with effort and perseverance, you can find relief and improve your quality of life.

Remember, you are not alone on this path. Consult your healthcare professional for advice and support, and rely on your loved ones for comfort and understanding. Celebrate minor triumphs along the way, such as eating a meal without discomfort or discovering a new favorite recipe that calms your digestive system.

Above all, be nice to yourself. Healing takes time, and setbacks are an expected part of the process. Continue to make positive adjustments in your food and lifestyle, and believe that each step you take will get you closer to long-term relief from acid reflux.

If this book has helped you manage your acid reflux, please consider providing a good review to share your experience with others. Your comment is vital, and it may encourage other seniors to embark on their own journey to better digestive health.

*Thank you for letting me be a part of your wellness journey. May your journey be full of comfort, vigor, and joy.*

*Warm Regards.*

*Christiana White.*

www.ingramcontent.com/pod-product-compliance
Lightning Source LLC
Chambersburg PA
CBHW081808250726
48653CB00010B/3845